Fertility: Family Planning:

Pregnancy Guide to Ovulation, Conception, Get Pregnant & Making Babies

Kristina Duclos

Getting Pregnant Fast Guide

Everything You Need to Know to Optimize Ovulation and Get Pregnant Faster

Kristina Duclos

Image courtesy of imagerymajestic / FreeDigitalPhotos.net

Table of Contents

Introduction

I want to thank you and congratulate you for purchasing the book, *'Getting Pregnant Fast Guide: Everything You Need to Know to Optimize Ovulation and Get Pregnant Faster.'*

There are a million of couples out there who are trying to get pregnant for a long time. Hence, if you are one of this million, remember that you are not alone! This reference book is going to help you!

It is true that it takes time to conceive a child in the womb. Being fertile at the right moment is not an easy proposition. There are other concerns that you have to take into consideration. As such, everybody advises you that it would be very important to exercise patience. According to them, getting pregnant is not similar to turning on the switch of the light bulb. This is not untrue. However, patience, although a good and solid advice, may not be enough.

The reason for this is that there are many factors that determine whether you will get pregnant in this month or not. The major factors are your health, ovulation and the sexual methods that you use. In this book, you will know how to optimize your chances of getting pregnant by properly caring for your health and nutrition, by tracking your ovulation, and by engaging in efficient sexual methods.

This book contains the most comprehensive optimization techniques of getting pregnant in order to help you in your personal goals. The goal of this book is to provide the reader with techniques, and strategies that they can readily perform. As such, the author of this book has made it possible to create a getting pregnant fast reference book that provides a good working knowledge of the fundamental concepts that is highly practical, instead of passive and abstract. Unnecessary jargon, together with vague terms and concepts, are avoided in order to make it simple and easy to apply. Moreover, effort has been done to make the getting pregnant fast reference book as intuitive and easy to learn as possible.

All in all, the methods that are outlined in this book will give you increased chances in getting pregnant soon. In fact, this book will provide you with the most sophisticated and efficient knowledge in terms of proper ovulation, nutrition and sexual methods that is already used by most health care professionals!

Thanks again for purchasing this book, I hope you enjoy it! Please take some time to stop by and LIKE our Facebook page: https://www.facebook.com/joypublishing

With gratitude,

Kristina Duclos

Chapter 1

The Fundamental Principles of Ovulation and Getting Pregnant

In this chapter you will learn:

- Understanding Ovulation

    o   Basics of Ovulation

    o   Ovulation Facts

    o   Ovulation: Does it occur before or after your period?

- Fertile Window

- The Fertile Phase of Your Cycle

- Signs of Ovulation

Understanding Ovulation

To put it simply, there is a 12 to 24 hour period when a fertile egg cell can be fertilized by a sperm cell. This is called the window of conception. Take note however, that the window of conception (12 to 24 hour period) is *not* the only time when conception (and getting pregnant) is possible. Do you want to know why? The reason is that unlike the fertile egg cell that is only available for a limited time, the sperm is available at any period of time. In fact, a sperm cell can live and survive inside the female uterus for up to five days! This is the reason why conception (and getting pregnant) is possible even after the window of conception. This concept will be further discussed in the latter part of this chapter and in chapter 2.

Understanding ovulation and the window of conception is the most important knowledge in getting pregnant fast. The reason for its importance lies in the fact that: By having a good working knowledge of the fundamental principles of ovulation and the window of conception, you and your partner will be able to know when is the best time to engage in sexual intercourse in order to get pregnant. In other words, you and your partner will be able to schedule the engagement in sexual intercourse in a time that is the most optimal for conception or getting pregnant.

Basics of Ovulation

Scientifically speaking, ovulation is the point in time when a female egg cell was released from the ovary. Afterwards, the female egg cell will travel down the fallopian tube where it will wait its turn to be fertilized by a sperm cell. Now, during the period of ovulation, if an egg cell that has been successfully been fertilized by a sperm cell, the lining of the uterine wall will thicken in order to give way to pregnancy.

Ovulation Facts

1. The cycle of ovulation usually alternates between the two ovaries

2. It is not impossible for a female to have ovulation even if she was not able to experience her period during a month

3. Light bleeding may happen during the cycle of ovulation

4. Only 1 egg cell is usually released from the ovary during each ovulation cycle

5. The egg cell will be available for fertilization for a period of 12 to 24 hours.

Ovulation: Does it occur before or after your Period?

One of the most frequently asked question is where ovulation occurs before or after the period. Technically speaking, ovulation should happen around the 14 day period immediately preceding your period. Does this mean that the best time to engage in sexual intercourse is on day 14 before your period?

Take note that this period assumes that your monthly cycle is 28 days. However, it is important to take into consideration that no woman is similar to any other! Therefore, it will be possible that your monthly cycle is 32 instead of 28 days.

In other words, there is even a slim chance that ovulation will happen on day 14 of your monthly cycle. As such, your chance of getting pregnant during that time is also slim.

Fertile Window

The best time to engage in sexual intercourse is solely dependent on the cycle of your ovulation. According to a recent research conducted by experts in physiology and female anatomy, for each cycle, the chance of getting pregnant is for exactly 6 days. This is the Critical 6 Day Fertile Window. The Critical 6 Day Fertile Window includes the time that the female egg cell is immediately available for fertilization (for 12 to 24 hours) and the 5 days immediately preceding ovulation.

Outside the Critical 6 Day Fertile Window, the chances of getting pregnant is very slim. In other words, knowing your Critical 6 Day Fertile Window is very important. According to the said study, the best chance of getting pregnant is at the following times in relation to the day of ovulation:

1. The day 2 days immediately preceding the day of ovulation;

2. The day immediately preceding the day of ovulation;

3. The day of ovulation itself.

The Fertile Phase of Your Cycle

The Fertile Phase of your cycle should not be confused with the Critical 6 Day Fertile Window. The Fertile Phase refers to the days in your ovulation cycle in which you may be within the Critical 6 Day Fertile Window. In other words, the Critical 6 Day Fertile Window is inside the fertile phase. For most women, the fertile phase happens between Day 6 and Day 21 of your cycle (a total of 16 days). However, it would be important to take into consideration that if you have a history of cycles that are highly irregular, your fertile phase may be much longer than that mentioned. If that is the case, you can use the signs of ovulation discussed below in order to help you determine the time of your ovulation.

Signs of Ovulation

The cycle of ovulation differs from one woman to another. As such, the cycle of ovulation of your mother (during her younger years), your sister or your friend will not be similar to yours. However, the biological changes that happen to women during the cycle of ovulation is fairly similar for each woman. Therefore, the signs of ovulation are consistent. These signs of ovulation are more commonly referred to as the symptoms of ovulation.

Basically, there are two types of symptoms of ovulation:

1. Primary symptoms of ovulation;

2. Secondary symptoms of ovulation.

On the one hand, primary symptoms of ovulation refer to that type of symptoms that are experienced by all women and can readily be spotted. The primary symptoms of ovulation are the following:

- Basal body temperature spike

- Cervical mucus becomes more slippery

- Cervical position becomes more firm

On the other hand, secondary symptoms of ovulation refer to that type of symptoms that may not be experienced by all women. In addition, these symptoms are not easily recognizable. The secondary symptoms of ovulation are the following:

- Bloating

- Increased sexual urge or libido

- Sense of smell are heightened

- Sense of touch are heightened

- Sense of taste are heightened

- Light spotting

- Tenderness of the breasts

- Cramping

- Pain on one side

Remember that as a woman, you may or may not notice the secondary symptoms of ovulation. Not noticing the secondary symptoms is perfectly fine. However, if you do notice these types of symptoms, you can have an additional guide in order to track your ovulation. Tracking of the cycle of ovulation is discussed thoroughly in the succeeding chapter, A Guide on Optimizing Your Chances of Getting Pregnant by Tracking Your Ovulation.

Chapter 2

A Guide on Optimizing Your Chances of Getting Pregnant by Tracking Your Ovulation

In this chapter you will learn:

- Key Concepts in Getting Pregnant

- The Simple Calendar Method

- Natural Family Planning (Fertility Awareness)

- Ovulation Tests and Monitors

Key Concepts in Getting Pregnant

Once you know your period of ovulation, it will be relatively easier for you and your partner to create a schedule on when to engage in sexual intercourse. The problem however is that tracking your ovulation will not be easy, if not difficult. In this chapter, different ways on how to track your ovulation are outlined in order to help you reach your goal of getting pregnant fast.

However, keep in mind that it would be your and your partner's job to preserve the spontaneity and romance in your loving relationship. The reason is that many couples who have been struggling to get pregnant in the past have made sex more of a chore than an expression of mutual love and care. As such, it would be crucial to avoid thinking that you are engaging in sexual intercourse for the sole reason of getting pregnant.

As previously stated in the first chapter, the 12 to 24 hour window of conception is the period when your fertile egg cell will be ready to be fertilized by the sperm cell of your partner. Also, it has been stated that the sperm cell of your partner can live inside your uterus for a period of 5 days. This is the main reason why the Critical 6 Day Fertile Window is 6 days and not 12 to 24 hours. Now, the question is this: How can you take advantage of this fact?

Remember that there is a greater chance of conception and getting pregnant when:

- The sperm cell is waiting inside the female uterus for the egg cell (during the Critical 6 Day Fertile Window); compared when

- It is the egg cell that is waiting to be fertilized by the sperm cell (during the exact point of ovulation).

Do you know the reason? It is because the first option provides you and your partner with a lot more flexibility and leeway (6 days) as compared to trying to precisely time your engagement in sexual intercourse at the exact point of ovulation (12 to 24 hours).

You may now be asking on what are the ways on which you can efficiently track your ovulation. To put it simply, there are 2 basic ways on which you can track your ovulation:

1. Using the calendar method (will be discussed shortly)

2. Using the primary and secondary symptoms of ovulation (as discussed in the first chapter).

Apart from the calendar method and the symptoms of ovulation, there are alternative ways and methods in which you can track your ovulation. These alternative ways are:

- Natural Family Planning (Fertility Awareness; and

- Ovulation Tests and Monitors.

Both of these methods will be discussed below.

The Simple Calendar Method

Actually, there are a lot of calendar based methods that are specifically designed to determine the exact time of ovulation. These methods include the following:

- ❖ Standard Days Method

- ❖ Modified Standard Days Method

- ❖ Rhythm Method

- ❖ The Simple Calendar Method

The Standard Days Method, Modified Standard Days Method, and the Rhythm Method are not discussed in this work because they are complicated in the sense that they will require you to make calculations solely based on the tracking period that you did for several months at a time. Also, most of them are based on flawed assumptions. In other words, should you use them, there is a chance that you might be missing out on key opportunities for getting pregnant each month. As such, it is believed that the simple calendar method is the best calendar method that you can use in order to determine the exact point or time of your ovulation.

In Simple Calendar Method, you will simply count 10 days immediately succeeding the first day you bleed. The first day you bleed refers to the first day of your monthly menstruation cycle. Now, what you will do is to engage in sexual intercourse with your partner every other day until the 21st day of your menstruation cycle.

In this way, you will be able to take advantage of the Critical 6 Day Fertile Window. In addition, there will also be some 'leeway days'. The reason for the existence of the 'leeway days' is that the exact point or time of your ovulation may vary from one month to another. Hence, taking into consideration the aforementioned variances, it would be prudent to include some 'leeway days' into the Critical 6 Day Fertile Window.

Natural Family Planning (Fertility Awareness)

Natural Family Planning refers to the practice of determining the exact day of your ovulation through the following means:

- Monitoring your temperature using a basal thermometer; and

- Checking your cervical mucus

The purpose of monitoring your temperature using a basal thermometer is that such thermometer is very sensitive and will reflect a sudden increase in your temperature that happens during the day of your ovulation.

The purpose of checking your cervical mucus is that during the period of your ovulation, the cervical mucus becomes more slippery, wet, and elastic. In addition, you will notice that your cervical mucus has the capability of being stretched between your fingers if you pull them apart and press them together. Some women described the texture of the cervical mucus during the period of ovulation as similar to egg whites.

Ovulation Tests and Monitors

Ovulation Tests and Monitors refers to a series test strips which is used in order to determine the surge of Luteinizing Hormone (LH) in your urine immediately preceding the period of ovulation.

The best thing about using these Ovulation Tests and Monitors is that the surge of Luteinizing Hormone (LH) in your urine happens during the 3 days immediately preceding the period of ovulation. As already stated, this 3 day window is one of the best times for conception. The reason for this is that such 3 day period is *well within* the Critical 6 Day Fertile Window. In other words, by using the ovulation test and monitor strips, it will be relatively easier for you and your partner to schedule the time for engagement in sexual intercourse that has the best chance of conceiving a child!

Chapter 3

A Guide on Optimizing Your Chances of Getting Pregnant Through Sexual Methods

In this chapter you will learn:

- The Best Sexual Position to Increase the Chances of Getting Pregnant

- Frequency of Sexual Intercourse

- Timing of Sexual Intercourse

- Things That You Should Never Do

The Best Sexual Position to Increase the Chances of Getting Pregnant

You might be wondering, "Is there a correct and incorrect way in performing sexual intercourse?" The answer is a simple no. The fact of the matter is you can get pregnant with *any* sexual position. Remember that as long as the sperm cell meets the egg cell, conception is possible. In other words, as long as there is contact of the semen of your partner in your vagina, there is a chance of getting pregnant. As such, it may be more important for you to use your efforts in the making sure that the sperm cells of your partner are of utmost health.

However, if there is one sexual position that you can use in order to maximize the chances of getting pregnant – such sexual position is the 'missionary style' where your partner will be on top and while you are lying on the bed. The reason is that the semen will be in the best position to reach the innermost part of your vagina (your uterus) immediately after ejaculation. In addition, it would be even better if you can use the modified missionary style sexual position where your partner is on top while you are lying on the bed with your legs elevated over his shoulders. In this way, you will be greatly aided by gravity and it also allows for deepest penetration.

Thus, the 'missionary style,' as far as the other sexual positions are concerned, is the best sexual position to increase your chances of getting pregnant.

Frequency of Sexual Intercourse

The frequency of sexual intercourse is an important component of getting pregnant fast. The reason for this is that the frequency of sexual intercourse will directly affect the quantity and quality of your partner's sperm cells. To put it simply:

1. On the one hand, if the frequency of sexual intercourse is too low (i.e., over the span of one week, he was not able to ejaculate), the seminal fluid will be filled with a good number of damaged and dead sperm cells.

2. On the other hand, if the frequency of sexual intercourse is too high (i.e., over the span of one week, he was able to ejaculate every day), the seminal fluid will be filled with a good number of immature and young sperm cells.

In both cases, the seminal fluid will not be as effective in conceiving a child. The recommended frequency of sexual intercourse is every other day during your fertile phase. In this way, you and your partner will be able to maximize the full quality and quantity of the sperm cells that is potent for fertilization. If you and your partner cannot manage to have sexual intercourse every other day, then every three days will also be optimal.

Timing of Sexual Intercourse

The time when men are most fertile is during the morning after a good sleep the night before. Hence, it is during the morning when men have the most quantity of sperm cells available. Therefore, it would make sense to schedule your sexual intercourse during the morning immediately after waking up.

Things That You Should Never Do

There are 5 things that you should never do if you want to optimize the chances of conception and getting pregnant. These are the following:

1. Avoid taking medications such as antihistamines. Although antihistamines might solve your problem with colds, it was found that they can also dry up your cervical mucus. Dry cervical mucus will prevent the sperm cells from reaching your uterus.

2. Do not engage in sexual intercourse while in a hot tub. Remember that high temperature quickly kills sperm cells.

3. Most commercially available lubricants today contain spermicides. As such, you have to avoid using them. However, should you really need lubricants, make sure that they do not contain spermicides by reading their contents.

4. Do not engage in sexual intercourse while bathing. Extreme temperatures, together with soap can kill the sperm cells.

5. Remind your partner that he should avoid using the laptop before engaging in sexual intercourse. The sperm cells are going to get killed from the heat of the laptop when placed near the groin area. However, should he really need to make use of the laptop, make sure that he puts the laptop on the table instead onto his lap.

Chapter 4

A Comprehensive Health and Nutrition Checklist during Conception

In this chapter you will learn:

- Nutrition and its importance

- Foods that you need to avoid

- Foods that you need to consume

Nutrition and its importance

When couples are trying to get pregnant, one of the questions that they frequently ask is: "Are there any foods that I can consume in order to help me get pregnant faster?" The answer is yes. Conversely, there are foods that you should avoid if you really want to get pregnant faster.

Good nutrition is synonymous with fertility. Therefore, eating well-balanced meals, eating the right kinds of foods, and avoiding the wrong kinds of foods will provide you with good health.

One of the best ways to increase the likelihood of getting pregnant is to invest in your health and well-being. Remember that a healthy body will enable you to do things that you want. One of those is trying to get pregnant. Conversely, if you are not presently healthy, your chances of getting pregnant may be low. In addition your good health at the time of conception will enhance the health and wellness of your future child in your womb.

Foods that you need to avoid

1. Caffeine

-   According to research, caffeine can effectively lower your fertility by 27%.

-   Apart from lowering your fertility, caffeine also hinders your body from absorbing essential nutrients such as calcium and iron.

2. Red Meat

-   According to research, red meat can effectively cause endometriosis. As such, red meat is a risk in lowering your levels of fertility.

-   In other words, it would be beneficial to limit your intake of red meat as much as possible.

3. Processed Foods

-   Many commercial processed foods today actually contain a lot of preservatives, artificial hormones and even pesticides. As such, apart from causing obesity, processed foods are very harmful by significantly decreasing the levels of your hormonal health.

-   Therefore you should avoid eating chips, frozen meals, cookies and other related food items such as hotdogs, bacon and sausage.

-   Instead, you should consume foods that are organic. This includes fresh vegetables and fruits.

4. Soy Products

• According to recent studies, products that are based on soy have been consistently shown to significantly diminish the sperm counts in men. The culprit is the isoflavone compound called Genistein. Genistein are seen to slow and destroy the sperm cells inside the human body.

• As such, you should ask your partner to avoid (at least while you are trying to get pregnant) products that are based on soy such as edmame, soy milk and tofu.

5. Simple Carbohydrates and Refined Sugars

• One of the reasons why simple carbohydrates and refined sugars must be avoided is that these kinds of foods cause weight gain and obesity. Remember that couples who are overweight are definitely less fertile compared to their slimmer counterparts.

• In addition, simple carbohydrates and refined sugars also cause your body to use up more nutrients in order to process them.

• As such, you should avoid eating foods such as sweets, sugar, white flour, white pastas, and other refined grains.

6. Bad Fats

• It is important to take into consideration that there are two kinds of fats – the good fats and the bad fats. Good fats are the kinds of fats that you should not avoid such as mono unsaturated fats found in olive oil.

• On the other hand, the fats that you should avoid are the bad fats. Bad fats are consistently found to decrease the levels of your fertility. Bad fats are:

  • partially hydrogenated fats (trans fats) found in processed foods; and

21

- saturated fats found in red meat

Foods That You Need to Consume

1. Water

- Water is very important to enable your organs to function more effectively. This is because water have a specific mechanism to help deliver the nutrients that you intake from food toward the rest of your body.

- In addition, remember that hormones are very important in pregnancy. It is consistently found by science that water causes hormonal balance throughout the body.

- Water also helps clear out the toxins out of your system.

2. Complex Carbohydrates

- Complex carbohydrates have nutrients that are favorable for pregnancy. In addition, complex carbohydrates also have fiber that is known to effectively remove the toxins out of your body.

- As such, remember to always consume carbohydrates such as brown rice, whole grain cereals, whole grain pasta, and vegetables.

3. Protein

- Protein is a nutrient that has a mechanism that contributes significantly in the production of hormones. As you now, hormones are very important in getting pregnant.

- The most healthy type of proteins are those found in foods such as oily fish, white meat, nuts, beans, seeds, and fresh eggs.

4. Whole Milk

- According to recent studies, drinking whole milk significantly increases the levels of fertility in women. According to the same research, women who drank at least 2 glasses of whole milk during the period of ovulation are 70% more likely to get pregnant.

- The reason, according to the researchers, is that whole milk contains natural hormones that boost the fertility of women.

- As such, it would be beneficial if you consume whole milk while you are trying to get pregnant.

Conclusion

Thank you again for purchasing this book!

Most likely, this getting pregnant fast reference book has provided you with ideas on how to increase your odds of getting pregnant soon!

I hope this book was able to help you to know the optimized techniques and strategies with respect to ovulation, nutrition and sexual methods with the goal of helping you get pregnant fast!

The next step you have to take in getting pregnant fast is to apply this knowledge every day (with respect to nutrition and the sexual methods) and every menstrual cycle (with respect to ovulation). Be sure to re-read it on a regular basis to remind yourself and make the most of it in your life! Soon enough, you will have that 'positive' result on your pregnancy test!

Finally, if you enjoyed this book and found it meaningful, please take the time to share your thoughts and post a positive review on Amazon. I greatly appreciate your time and effort.

I would love for you to share your experiences, stories and encouragements with me. My email address is

kristinaducloskindle@gmail.com

In addition, please remember to check out our Facebook page in order to find other resources and upcoming promotions:

https://www.facebook.com/joypublishing

Sincerely, Kristina Duclos

How to Predict Your Baby Gender

Guide to Fertility and Achieving the Baby Gender of Your Dreams

Kristina Duclos

Table Of Contents

Introduction

Dear Reader,

Thank you for purchasing *"How to Predict Your Baby Gender: Guide to Fertility and Achieving the Baby Gender of Your Dreams."* I feel so privileged to share my years of knowledge and experience with you in this informational and practical book.

I am the mother of a toddler and have personal experience with baby gender prediction techniques. I was successful in predicting the gender of my baby girl the moment I found out I was pregnant: over 15 weeks before any ultrasound test! I only officially confirmed her gender when she was born. During those eight months, I was confident that I was having a girl; I even went as far as purchasing a few butterfly and flower decorations for her nursery.

My hope is that through this book you will apply these prediction techniques to your own experience and find the same success that I did. Share my journey of birth control and pregnancy with me. Afterwards, learn the techniques for predicting your baby's gender. Finally, apply the techniques in your own life to create your own story. Even though Mother Nature will always make her plans, we are still able to swing the decision in a more favorable direction.

Please take some time to stop by and LIKE our Facebook page:

https://www.facebook.com/joypublishing

Enjoy,

Kristina Duclos

Chapter 1 - How It All Started: My Personal Journey

I easily get excited and passionate when talking about baby gender prediction techniques. I love sharing the information with anyone who will listen. Furthermore, I love impressing people with my own success of predicting my daughter's gender. This knowledge and experience that I gained about predicting baby gender originally came from a fantastic fertility awareness book that changed my life: Taking Charge of Your Fertility by Toni Weschler.

I was first introduced to the concepts of baby gender prediction and fertility awareness when I was switching from the birth control pill to some kind of natural method. I wasn't thrilled with the birth control pill. I believe that it altered my personality and made me feel "crazy." I was originally planning to switch to a different pill until I started reading Toni Weschler's book. It forever changed my attitude towards birth control and convinced me of the benefits of a more natural approach.

As I learned more about the intricacies of the female body, I developed a deep respect and awe for how the female body was built. At this point in time, I knew that I no longer wanted to use the birth control pill, even if I found one that was a better fit. On the contrary, I wanted to experience the ups and downs of my fertility cycle the way nature intended it to be. No more pills or synthetic hormones for me.

Once I taught myself how to read my body's fertility signs, I discovered the fascinating facts about baby gender prediction. I soon got pregnant and had the opportunity to interpret these facts in my own pregnancy. Although I never confirmed my baby's gender until after she was born, I knew her gender from day one based on the gender prediction techniques. It was as clear as day that I was having a girl.

Chapter 2 - Why Fertility Awareness and Not Some Other Natural Method?

Before I was ready to get pregnant, I needed to find a birth control method that I was satisfied with. During my journey to find something natural, I considered a few options: IUDs, condoms and withdrawal. As soon as I read Toni Wechler's book, I knew that natural birth control was the way for me. I had enough respect for my cycle that I no longer wanted to manipulate it.

IUD

One natural birth control option was the IUD (intrauterine device). In addition to the synthetic hormone releasing IUD, there is a non-hormonal version that uses copper. This is the option available to those who don't want the chemicals in their body.

After I did some research on the copper IUD, I soon discovered the process involved in preventing a woman from becoming pregnant. The copper from the IUD either kills the sperm before it fertilizes the egg; or if an egg is fertilized, the copper does not allow the egg to implant itself in the uterine lining. This information did not sit well with me and became too ethical. I disliked the idea of a little fertilized egg floating around my uterus, not able to attach itself in order to continue to grow. Consequently, this form of natural birth control was axed from my list.

Condoms

Condoms were the next option. Not a particular favorite of my husband. We agreed that condoms or abstinence would be used during my times of fertility. We were free to go without condoms during my infertile windows of time.

Withdrawal

The withdrawal method was just a ridiculous option. Anyone who uses the withdrawal method is uneducated about the male and female body. They also soon become parents. The reason why the withdrawal method doesn't work is because of the "pre-cum" that is released prior to a full ejaculation. If a woman is in her fertile phase, that "pre-cum" is sufficient enough to get the woman pregnant. We weren't taking any chances with that.

Chapter 3 - Pregnancy Achieved. A Baby Girl It Will Be.

I followed the Fertility Awareness birth control method for over two years before I was ready to get pregnant. Once I started trying to get pregnant, it didn't take long to conceive. After the first month, I was successful! The main key to my success was that I knew exactly when I was fertile and I used that window of time very wisely. During that fertile phase is when I focused the most on the timing of intercourse.

Predicting the gender of the baby was easy as well. I used my knowledge of ovulation timing and the characteristics of sperm to determine that I was having a girl. As I charted my fertility, intercourse and ovulation, I noticed that there were several days between the day of intercourse and the day of ovulation. This charted information gave me the certainty that I was having a girl and the unlikelihood of having a boy.

Chapter 4 - The Beauty of the Female Cycle

It was discovering the rhythms of the female cycle that stole me over to the natural side of birth control and family planning. I discovered beauty in the intricacies of the female cycle and gained a deep respect for the complexities of how her body was made.

Each month, the female actually prepares to get pregnant. That's what she was designed to do. When a woman is not successful, the body disposes of all its hard work, in the form of a period, and then starts again. Then again, and again, every month.

This may be contrary to what you're used to thinking about the female body. You may see the female body as infertile every month, through the display of a period. Once she gets pregnant, her period disappears for 9 plus months. It almost appears to me as if the female cycle is "dead" each month until there is finally a "life" in the form of a pregnancy.

Opposite to that concept is the idea that the female body attempts "life" each month and then gets rid of the "dead" stuff before it prepares for "life" again. This is a much more beautiful way of seeing the female cycle. It is actually designed to give life. This purpose is consistent with the caring and nurturing nature of woman.

Here's how it works in a simple explanation:

The female's cycle starts with three to fives days of menstruation. This is when the body sheds the lining of the uterus that has been built up over the last couple weeks. Once the lining is removed in the form of a period, the body starts building up with the estrogen hormone.

Estrogen continues to build and increase in the body, preparing several eggs (ova) in the ovaries for ovulation. Finally, during ovulation, a single egg (ovum) is released from one ovary and starts its journey down the fallopian tube. The ovum continues its journey down the fallopian tube towards the uterus, seeking to be united with a single sperm. Estrogen drops and progesterone spikes, which is the signal that ovulation has been achieved.

If the ovum is successful in obtaining fertilization, the body will send out a pregnancy hormone, human chorionic gonadotropin (hCG), to signal to the body to continue the production of progesterone. This progesterone is needed to build up and maintain the uterine lining for the fertilized ovum during the remainder of the pregnancy.

If, however, fertilization is not obtained, the pregnancy hormone will not be release. Therefore, progesterone will drop and the uterine lining will begin to detach from the uterine wall. The lining descends down the vagina, along with the unfertilized ovum, and exits the body in the form of a period. Afterwards, the whole cycle starts again with the build up of estrogen.

It's such a beautiful symphony every month: the ups and downs of estrogen and progesterone, both serving a different purpose. One builds up life. The other maintains life.

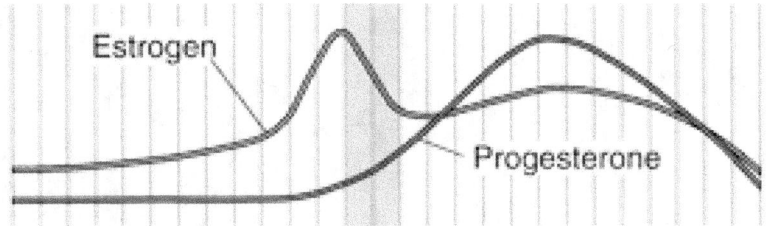

www.merckmanuals.com

Chapter 5 - The Power of Knowing Your Cycle

The quickest way to fire me up is to start talking to women about the value and importance of being educated about their fertility cycle. There is so much power in charting the female cycle and knowing the ins and outs.

Below is a list of the reasons why a woman should be familiar with her personal fertility cycle:

1. Avoiding an unwanted pregnancy

2. Planning a wanted pregnancy

3. No bush beating

4. Knowing right from wrong

5. No pregnancy test needed

6. Due date accuracy

Avoiding an Unwanted Pregnancy

When a woman charts her fertility cycle, she knows when she is fertile and when she isn't. Using this information, the woman can abstain from intercourse or use a back up method during the days of fertility in order to prevent an unwanted pregnancy.

Planning a Wanted Pregnancy

Once a woman is ready to get pregnant, the knowledge of fertile and infertile periods of time has already been established. The opposite strategy used for preventing a pregnancy would be practiced: focusing on intercourse during the fertile window. A woman is actually only fertile for 24 hours, the lifespan of the ovum. As a result, the pressure to get pregnant is taken off during the other 29ish days of the month.

There are many couples who have being trying to get pregnant for months or even years. Some have resolved to be infertile and have had to pursue other methods for conception. However, many of the couples who have been unsuccessful with getting pregnant are still perfectly fertile. The problem is that they are not educated about their window of fertility and then utilizing that information for their benefit. They are essentially "hitting and missing" each month. Instead of just aimlessly having intercourse each month, they need to be strategically planning their intercourse for when it counts: during their window of fertility.

No Bush Beating

If a woman were to discover that she is having difficulty getting pregnant, she can avoid beating around the bush with her doctor to figure out why she isn't being successful. Instead of having several variables that could be contributing to infertility, the variables can be narrowed down to one through the charting of the female cycle.

For example, a woman notices that she is ovulating but her luteal phase is short She many actually be getting pregnant but the phase of progesterone is too short to maintain the uterine wall. Therefore, the fertilized ovum is being flushed out with the rest of the uterine lining during her period. The woman can now take this information to the doctor and get the specific help she needs for the specific problem in her cycle. That just eliminated a slough of testing that could have been completely unnecessary.

Knowing Right From Wrong

Knowing what's "right" and "wrong," or normal and abnormal about the female cycle is crucial to a female's health. A woman uneducated about her body may think that every little leak or discoloration is "bad." As a result, she is rushing off to the doctor to get her next round of medication to fix the problem that isn't even a problem. Surely the doctor would be smart enough to not misdiagnose her.

A woman would save herself a lot of wasted time and stress if she knew what was "right" about her body. There is no need to study what's "wrong" since there is an endless list of possibilities. She only needs to educate herself about what is "right." Then what's "wrong" will be obvious.

Consider the following analogy: a banker filtering through a wad of counterfeit bills. The banker only needs to know what an authentic dollar bill feels and looks like. If she were to take the time to learn about all the different counterfeit bills available, she would be wasting her time. There are an endless number of varieties with new ones being created all the time. There is no way she would be able to keep up with all the different forms of counterfeits. Consequently, the best use of her time is to determine the qualities of an authentic bill. Therefore, as she quickly sifts through the bills with her fingers, she can immediately pick out the fakes.

The same is with our female body. When we know what is "right," we are quick to pick out what is "wrong" and then fix it in whatever way necessary.

No Pregnancy Test Needed

I had the privilege of discovering when I was pregnant before I even took a pregnancy test. The reason for my knowing was due to the progesterone spike after ovulation. This period of time is called the luteal phase (mentioned previously). During this phase of the female cycle, progesterone remains high to maintain the uterine lining. If pregnancy is not achieved, progesterone drops, the lining is shed and the cycle starts again. A typical luteal phase is approximately 12 to 16 days if there is the absence of the pregnancy hormone.

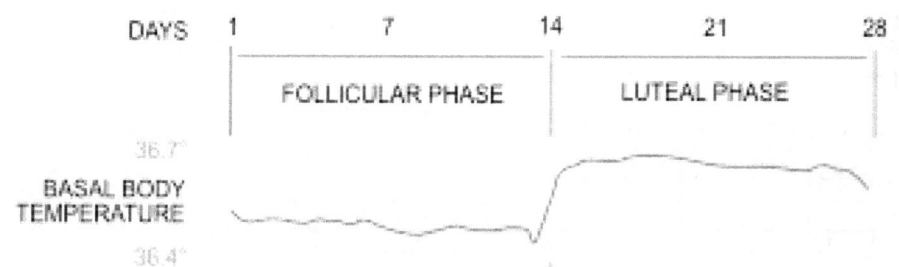

www.merckmanuals.com

However, if conception is successful, the pregnancy hormone communicates to the progesterone to continue producing. This luteal phase extends from the typical 12 to 16 days to 18 days and more. This was the key to discovering that I was pregnant. I was highly confident that I was pregnant when I charted more than 18 days during my luteal phase. I confirmed with a pregnancy test, two times, and was right!

Due Date Accuracy

Most ovulation predictor kits or due date calendars assume that women have a typical 28 day cycle with ovulation occurring on day 14. However, this isn't always the case with a lot of women. As a result, inaccurate due dates can be calculated because of a longer or shorter cycle.

In my situation, I had my due date pushed back several days because I knew that I did not ovulate on day 14. I ovulated a few days later based on my charted information. My typical cycle was 32 days rather than 28. Therefore, I asked my prenatal care provider to reevaluate my due date.

My information was accurate when I had my dating ultrasound at 7 weeks. The sonogram confirmed that the embryo was measuring younger than the expected age. Therefore, my due date was moved back a few days.

It's important to have an accurate due date because doctors use this information to determine whether a baby is "late" after 40 weeks of pregnancy. They will then decide if a woman needs to be induced or not. Being induced is a decision to take seriously. If induction could have been avoided because of a more accurate due date, then all the better for the mother and unborn baby. Perhaps the baby wasn't as "late" as the doctor thought it was. Maybe, it was actually right on time.

Chapter 6 - Figuring Out When You're Fertile

The body has 3 natural fertility signs that will help you know when you're fertile, if read correctly. These three signs are:

1. Basal Body Temperature

2. Cervical Fluid

3. Cervix Position

Basal Body Temperature

A woman's basal body temperature is determined when she awakes in the morning, before she even gets out of bed. Her basal temperature is low during the rise of estrogen until ovulation. After ovulation, the basal temperature spikes and remains high until the period starts. Or, conversely, remains high if pregnancy is achieved.

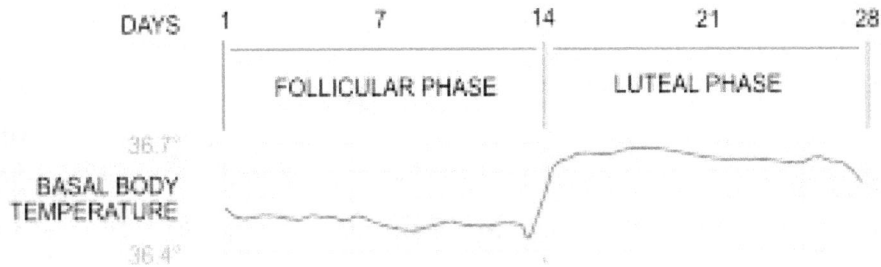

www.merckmanuals.com

The cause for the spike in temperature is due to the spike in progesterone. Since progesterone is a heat hormone, it emits heat. This stable spike in temperature is the indicator that ovulation has occurred.

The basal body temperature charting confirms a successful ovulation and pregnancy. It is only in hindsight that you can see the fertile windows of time. Therefore, it isn't as useful in helping determine when to time intercourse. That's when cervical fluid comes into play.

Cervical Fluid

The second fertility sign is the cervical fluid. The cervical fluid is used to indicate when a woman is fertile and infertile. The best way to notice your cervical fluid is by paying attention to your underwear when you go to the bathroom. I know some women are raised into thinking that they are "dirty" down there. But you are not. Remind yourself of the beauty of the female cycle and what it is preparing for each month.

During a woman's period, the cervical fluid released is the uterine lining (we all know what that looks like). Once the lining passes, the cervical fluid is dry. A piece of tissue does not slide smoothly along the exterior of the vulva when wiped. It is during this time (from the start of the period to the end of the dry phase) that a woman is infertile. During this phase of infertility, sperm can only live for a few hours in the vagina.

While the body is releasing estrogen, building towards ovulation, the cervical fluid changes from dry to sticky. It can appear white and gummy or can even look like rubber cement. This is a sign that the woman is starting to enter into the fertile phase. Be weary of this phase if you are trying to avoid getting pregnant.

The woman enters her fertile phase when her cervical fluid changes to an egg white consistency. The fluid looks clear and watery and is also incredibly stretchy. The woman may feel a slippery sensation when she walks. Furthermore, a tissue slides very freely along the exterior of the vulva when wiped. In this fertile condition, sperm can last up to 5 days! This cervical fluid is like a super highway for the sperm to reach the egg in the fallopian tube. The sperm adheres to this fluid and is able to travel quickly to its destination.

Knowing the characteristics of sperm is important during this fertile phase in order to help you predict your baby's gender. Since sperm can live in a fertile condition for up to 5 days, they can enter the body prior to ovulation and hang out until the ovum is released. This information can be used to decide whether you will have intercourse closer or further away from ovulation. The decision depends on whether a boy or girl is desired.

This is exactly how I knew that I was pregnant with a girl. I had intercourse six days before ovulation. The female sperm hung around until the ovum was released while the male sperm were already long gone. Then, a single female sperm was ready to fertilize the ovum at just the right time.

The day of ovulation is the peak of the fertile phase and the last day of the egg white cervical fluid.

If a woman really wants to be certain about her cervical fluid, she can insert her clean fingers into her vagina to remove some fluid from the base of the cervix. This can be tricky to do.

Cervix Position

The position of the cervix is the last fertility sign. It isn't as commonly used. Furthermore, it does require some probing around in your vagina to determine whether it is positioned high or low, open or closed. If the cervix is high and open, you are fertile. If it is low and closed, you are not. You can also tell sometimes when the woman is on top during intercourse. If a woman feels discomfort during penetration, the cervix is generally in the low position. Woman may use this sign to confirm if they are in their fertile phase.

Chapter 7 - Preparing for Pregnancy

Creating the life of another human being is incredible but also sobering. Your life will no longer be yours. You'll need to sacrifice your needs and wants for the needs of your baby. It is important for a woman to prepare for pregnancy in order to give her baby the best chance. There are five things a woman can do prior to conception to ensure she is healthy for pregnancy.

1. Exercise

2. Diet

3. Relaxation

4. Folic Acid

5. Ovulation Timing

Exercise

Pregnancy is physically demanding on a woman's body. The more she exercises, the better prepared she will be to not only carry the weight of the baby, but also to be successful during labor. It is said that a woman's body remembers her pre-pregnancy weight and can quickly return to that weight after the birth of her baby. It is also important to exercise during pregnancy so that a woman does not put on unnecessary weight that will only be harder to loose after the baby. Doctors recommend 30 minutes a day. It is important to keep the heart rate up during the physical activity.

Diet

Coupled with exercise is maintaining a healthy diet. The word diet is not used in the sense of restricting or limiting your food intake to loose weight. It is simply used in the manner of having a well-balanced diet of grains, fruits, vegetables, meat and alternatives and milk and alternatives. It is also important to maintain a healthy diet during pregnancy so the baby gets all the nutrients it needs for proper development.

Relaxation

It can be hard to get pregnant if a woman has a lot of stress in her life. Some woman can try getting pregnant for years simply because of the stress from trying to conceive. It is in a woman's best interest to find ways to relax in order to help her body achieve conception. Once a woman is pregnant, it is so critical to maintain the attitude of relaxation with activities such as yoga or reading. Stress can cause miscarriages or even affect the unborn fetus.

Folic Acid

At least one month prior to trying to conceive, a woman should take 400 mcg (micrograms) or .4 mg (milligrams) of folic acid. Research shows that taking folic acid reduces the chances of babies developing neural-tube defects such as spina bifida by at least 70% (Centers for Disease Control and Prevention). A woman should continue taking folic acid during her pregnancy.

Ovulation Timing

Part of the stress women encounter when trying to get pregnant is not knowing when they will ovulate. In order to reduce this stress, women can use a variety of techniques to help pin point when they are ovulating so they can optimize intercourse. The most popular technique is using an ovulation predictor kit.

Chapter 8 - Pregnancy Signs

Once a woman is trying to conceive, the wait to find out if she is pregnant can be torture. A pregnancy test is the most common tool a woman uses to determine if pregnancy was achieved. Using the Fertility Awareness Method, a woman can know she is pregnant well before taking a pregnancy test. When a woman charts her basal body temperature, she will know she is pregnant if her body maintains a high temperature for more than 18 days post ovulation. Regardless of whether a woman uses a pregnancy test or her basal body temperature, what are the pregnancy signs?

A Missed Period

A missed period is the most tell-a-tale sign that a woman is pregnant. When a woman conceives, her body produces the pregnancy hormone to inform the body that a conception was successful. This warning tells the body to not shed the lining it had been developing prior to ovulation. If a woman has just had a baby, the return of a period is not a sign that she has started ovulation. A woman can actually ovulate prior to receiving her period. Therefore, a woman should never wait for her period to return in order know that she has started her menstrual cycle again.

Implantation Spotting

Once an egg is fertilized, it travels to the uterus to plant itself in the uterus lining. Light bleeding can occur (about 10 days after ovulation) that is called implantation spotting. Some woman can mistaken this bleeding as their period and think they are safe from pregnancy. This is not the case at all. It is important to notice the difference between the spotting and a typical period. Spotting is lighter in flow with a pink or brownish color.

Tender Breasts

A woman's breasts or nipples can become incredibly tender when she is pregnant. They can also become more full and larger in size. The areola can start to darken as well.

Nausea

Nausea, or morning sickness, is another tell-a-tale sign of pregnancy. Although it is called morning sickness, it doesn't always occur in the morning. Some women have extreme cases of nausea to the point when they need to take medication to cope. Typically, nausea passes after the first trimester. Some women find the nausea reassuring that the embryo is still alive. Drinking ginger ale, eating crackers, putting a cool cloth behind the neck or taking B6 vitamins are a few of the ways to help alleviate the annoyance of nausea.

Fatigue

Feeling more tired or exhausted than usual is a common sign of pregnancy. The body has kicked into high gear in order to create another human being. As a result, a lot of the body's energy is being channeled into the embryo.

Excessive Urination

Frequent urination in the first trimester has a different cause than the third trimester. In the first trimester, there is an increase in blood volume and the size of the kidneys. These two factors influence the increased need to pee. In the third trimester, the growing uterus pushes on the bladder, causing it to empty itself more frequently.

Mild Ache in Lower Abdomen

If a mild ache, bloating or fullness is felt in the lower abdomen, a woman can be pregnant instead of having PMS. This feeling is from the implantation of the egg in the uterus lining.

Moodiness

Due to the dramatic increase in hormones, a woman may experience moodiness and irritation. Don't just chalk it up to PMS.

Chapter 9 - Reasons to Know the Gender of Your Baby

As soon as a woman shares with the world that she is pregnant, she'll get variations of the same question: "is it a boy or a girl?" Or, if it's early in the pregnancy, "are you going to find out the gender?"

People are always curious to know the sex of the baby. Before the age of technology, the gender of a baby was always left a mystery. Nowadays, the secrecy of the womb is being revealed due to the availability of technology, such as ultrasounds. While large populations of pregnant parents want to be surprised when their baby is born, they are quickly becoming the majority. About 9 out of 10 parents are interested in predicting their baby's gender.

There are a variety of reasons for this modern luxury of discovering the baby's gender. Fortunately, the gender selection techniques for predicting baby gender are safe, inexpensive and natural! They are best applied in the planning stages prior to pregnancy so the gender of choice can be better conceived.

Below are some of the many reasons why people want to discover the gender of their baby:

1. For those people who love to plan, it is an absolute must to discover the gender of the baby. These people need to buy all the baby's clothes and paraphernalia specific to its sex. Names are easier to pick and paint colors are easier to decide.

2. They already have one child and would like to know whether they need to save all their gender specific baby stuff or get rid of it.

3. They already have one or two children of one gender and are willing to have another child to gamble for the opposite gender. People that have two children of the same sex are way more likely to try for a third. People, who have one of each gender, are more likely to stop after two.

4. They prefer a particular gender due to cultural or religious reasons.

5. They simply just want to know.

How would you go about knowing or predicting the gender of your baby?

There are many ways to go about predicting your baby's gender. Some methods are more scientific for determining gender of baby during pregnancy, while others are just myths or old wives tales.

Medical Tests

  Genetic testing

  Ultrasound scans

Less Conventional Tests

  Needle or Wedding Ring Test

  Drano Test

  The Intelligender Gender Test

  Chinese Gender Calendar

Woman's Intuition

Old Wives Tales

Gender Myths and Gender Quiz

Semi-Scientific Tests

Baby's Heart Rate Test

Shettles Method

Fertility Awareness Method

Although we can't control nature, the gender selection techniques for predicting baby gender can be used to greatly increase the likelihood of achieving a particular gender. Similarly, we are unable to go to a store and pick out the baby boy or girl we want. However, we can use the predicting baby gender techniques listed in this ebook to tip the scales or increase the odds in our favour.

Chapter 10 - Common Medical Tests

Once pregnancy is achieved, women are limited to the ways they can determine the sex of their baby. Currently, genetic testing (CVS (chronionic villus sampling) and amniocentesis) and ultrasound scans are the only medical tests that can be conducted for discovering a baby's gender.

CVS (chronionic villus sampling) and amniocentesis have 99% accuracy for how to predict the baby's gender as early as 10 weeks. However, these methods pose a risk to your baby due to the long needle that is inserted inside your pregnant belly. Not only is there a risk of miscarriage for these two procedures, these tests are used for genetic information only. Therefore, doctors are not as likely to conduct these tests for the sole purpose of predicting baby gender.

Around a woman's 20 week mark, she is usually offered a routine ultrasound. At this point in the pregnancy, the baby's gender can often be clearly revealed. This procedure is the most common, safe and pain free. However, the results are not 100% accurate if the baby is not in the right position. Furthermore, you need to wait for 20 weeks, which can be agony!

Unfortunately, there are some ultrasound agencies that do not allow ultrasound technicians to reveal to the client the gender of the baby. The reason for this is to protect the unborn child from being aborted if the parents do not like the result. Depending on the area you live in, you may need to pay the ultrasound agency or go through your doctor to get the results you desire.

Chapter 11 - Less Conventional Tests

In addition to genetic testing and ultrasound scans, there are some less conventional methods for guessing your baby's gender. These tests include:

1. The Drano test

2. The well known needle or wedding ring test

3. The popular Chinese gender calendar

4. The Intelligender Gender test

5. A pregnant woman's intuition

6. Pre-Conception Diet

7. Key Test

8. Baby Activity

Drano Test

How to perform the Drano test:

You will need two tablespoons of Crystal Drano (not the liquid), rubber gloves, a disposable glass jar, safety glasses and an outdoor work space. First, collect a fresh urine sample (2 to 3 oz) when you wake up in the morning. Second, pour the Drano into the disposable glass jar. Add an equal amount of urine. Wait about 10 seconds. Predicting baby gender results: if the mix turns a dark brownish color within 10 seconds, it's a boy. If it does nothing for more than 10-15 seconds, it's a girl. While the Drano Test is a fun experiment to do, the results are open to interpretation and the test can be unsafe.

Warning: This test is dangerous for a pregnant woman to conduct due to the poisonous fumes. It works best after 4 months pregnant. However, this is not the time to be exposing yourself to potentially harmful fumes. Instead of putting yourself at risk, try a commercial product that works in the same way without being dangerous. The Intelligender Gender Test is an example of a commercial product available.

Needle or Wedding Ring Test

The needle or wedding ring test is a popular test that people like to try with their friends and family. It can be performed anywhere.

Attach a strand of hair or a piece of thread to a needle or wedding ring. Hold the needle or ring over the pregnant woman's belly while she is lying down. If the needle or ring swings in a strong circle, it's a girl. If it swings from side to side like a pendulum, it's a boy. As an alternative, you can dangle the needle or ring over the pregnant mom's wrist. Once again, even though this is a fun experiment to do with your friends and family, it is not 100% accurate due to human error from subliminal finger movements.

Chinese Gender Calendar

The Chinese gender calendar comes with many names: Chinese gender chart, Chinese gender predictor, Chinese pregnancy chart or calendar. It is an incredibly popular tool to use in predicting the baby's gender. Some people swear by it and others don't believe it at all.

The Chinese gender calendar, rumored to have been found 700 years ago in an ancient royal tomb near Beijing, China, is used for Chinese gender prediction. Some say the Chinese gender calendar is over 90% accurate. However, there are so many different charts available online, it is easy to get an inaccurate result. One Chinese gender calendar can say that you're having a boy and the other can say the opposite. The two most important numbers used for the Chinese gender calendar are the woman's age at conception and the month she conceived. The woman's age is based on her lunar age which is different than the Gregorian calendar system used in most parts of the world. The month the woman conceived is also based on the lunar calendar.

Note: the Chinese gender calendar is not based on science. Oddly, the Chinese gender prediction is based on the mother's age and the month of conception. How a woman's age has anything to do with ovulation and predicting a baby's gender seems unusual.

The Intelligender Gender Test

Similar to the Drano test, the Intelligender gender test also uses your morning urine for guessing the baby's gender. The urine is contained in a re-sealing container before the crystals are introduced. Once the urine meets the crystals, a chemical reaction will occur. Swirl the concoction around for a few seconds then place on a flat surface for about 10 seconds. An orange colour equals a girl. A murky greenish colour equals a boy. The test claims to be 90% accurate and you can use it as early as 10 weeks. Not only is the test safe, you don't come into contact with a smelly, potentially toxic substance. This test is preferred over the dangerous drano test. Mind you, it does cost a lot more money.

Woman's Intuition

Some women claim they have a gut feeling about their baby's gender when they first find out they are pregnant. Can a woman's intuition be a reliable form for guessing a baby's gender? According to a survey completed by the University of Arizona, "Women who claimed to have an intuition about the gender of their child made the right choice 70% of the time." It's quite impressive that women can have a sixth sense about the gender of their baby. Women will often report having dreams about the gender of their baby. While it does seem completely believable, the vivid dreams that women have can be due to the large surge of hormones in the woman's body caused by the pregnancy. (http://web.arizona.edu/~vas/intuit.htm).

Pre-Conception Diet

One popular myth for guessing baby gender is the pre-conception diet. This myth claims that what a woman eats before she conceives a baby can influence predicting baby gender. If a baby girl is desired, a diet full of dairy and magnesium rich foods (such as soy beans, nuts, and leafy green vegetables) should be consumed to most often. If a baby boy is desired, consume salty foods, red meat and soda pop. Furthermore, if you want a baby with lots of hair, eat spicy food frequently.

Note: this myth is not backed up by scientific research. The male sperm from the woman's partner is what determines the gender of a baby. The food a woman consumes before she gets pregnant has absolutely no correlation with the male sperm. However, the foods eaten may alter the pH balance in the woman and therefore influence the male sperm. Nevertheless, it is important to clarify that it is not what a woman eats that determines the sex of the baby. The male sperm does that. Furthermore, an excess amount of food in the diet would need to be consumed with still no guarantee. The result would be an out of balance diet with a risk of important nutrients being missed. Guessing baby gender is still a 50% chance. A well-balanced nutritious diet is recommended more than anything else.

Key Test

Another myth for predicting baby gender is the key test. Present a pregnant woman with a key, such as a house or car key. If the key is picked up from the narrow end (tip), the woman is pregnant with a baby girl. If the key is picked up from the wide end (base), the woman is pregnant with a baby boy. Take note that this myth is not backed up by scientific research. There is no logical connection between the gender of the baby and which end of the key the woman picks up. More often than not, it is just random chance like flipping a coin. Guessing baby gender is still a 50% chance.

Baby Activity

The extent a baby is active in the womb is a common myth for guessing baby gender. If the baby is active, then you are having a baby boy. Conversely, if there is minimal activity, then you are having a baby girl.

Note: this myth is not backed up by scientific research. Furthermore, it does not take into account the pregnant woman's perception. Depending on the woman's activity, whether she is racing around or relaxing, will contribute to the degree of fetal activity. Babies can be lulled to sleep when mothers are being physically active. Ironically, they tend to be active when the exhausted pregnant woman is trying to get sleep for the night. In addition, this myth uses the stereotype of males generally being more active than females. Predicting baby gender continues to be 50% accurate. (Some information referenced from www.babyzone.com, www.canadianliving.com and www.friendasap.com)

An Alternative

An alternative to these different tests are specific gender selection techniques for predicting baby gender, which are 100% safe and proven to work. Check out my testimonials due to the learned strategies from this ebook for predicting a baby's gender.

Baby Jesse

Nancy was excited to share with me that she was pregnant. When it was revealed that Nancy had intercourse the same night she ovulated, I knew immediately how to predict her baby's gender. It was clear that Nancy was having a boy since the male sperm was the first to arrive at the egg due to its fast "swimming" capabilities.

Baby Anna

Away in Mexico on a romantic wedding anniversary vacation, a night of a few drinks soon got out of hand. One thing led to the next and Mary and John had unprotected sex. Mary thought she was safe because she was at the tale end of her period. Using this information, I was able to learn how to predict the baby's gender using the concepts of male sperm characteristics and ovulation timing. What Mary didn't realize was that her body was preparing for ovulation shortly after her period. Her fertile cervical fluid was masked by the flow of her menstruation. The male sperm was long gone while the female sperm patiently waited for the ovum to arrive. The sperm was able to live inside the uterus for a few days because the conditions were favorable.

Baby Ella

Using the Fertility Awareness Method, I knew I was pregnant before even taking a pregnancy test. Since I was educated about when I had intercourse and when ovulation occurred, I knew how to predict the gender. The day of intercourse was six days before ovulation without any intercourse in between. It was clear that I was having a girl due to the male sperm being dead several days before the female sperm arrived at the ovum. I was so confident I was having a girl that I purchased pink girly decorations for the nursery months before my due date.

Chapter 12 - Old Wives Tales and Gender Quiz

When you're pregnant, you'll notice that people love to try and guess the gender of your baby. They'll come up with all sorts of predictions as to why they think you are having a boy or girl. Listed below are some popular old wives tales from around the world. Some of the myths from the gender quiz are more ridiculous than others. The funny thing is, only 50% of the guesses are right. Complete the following checklist:

You're more likely to be having a boy if...

- you're carrying low and out front (like a basketball)

- you barely had morning sickness in the first trimester

- your right breast is bigger than your left

- your pupils dilate when you look at yourself in the mirror for at least a minute

- you crave salty and sour food or protein (eg. cheese and meat)

- you have dry skin and your feet are more cold compared to before you were pregnant

- you combine your age at the time of conception with the number of the month you conceived and the resulting number is even

- your hair has become more full and shiny

- you are more prone to headaches

- your pillow faces the north direction when you sleep

- the hair on your legs has been growing faster

- you lie on your left side when sleeping

- you present your hands palm down when you are asked to show them

- you eat a clove of garlic and then the smell seeps out of your pores

- your previous child's first word was "dada"

- you were the more aggressive partner when you conceived

- your husband does not gain weight during your pregnancy

- your urine is bright yellow

- your areolas (the ring around your nipples) have gotten much darker

- you look better than ever

Add up your "yes" and "no" columns. According to the old wives tales, if you had more "yes's" than "no's" you are more likely having a boy.

You're more likely to be having a girl if...

- you're carrying high and all round (like a watermelon)

- your left breast is bigger than your right

- you crave sweet things, fruits or vegetables

- you are more moody than normal

- you had lots of morning sickness during the first trimester

- you present your hands palm up when you are asked to show them

- you have soft skin

- your pupils don't dilate when you look at yourself in the mirror for at least a minute

- your pillow faces the south direction when you sleep

- you lie on your right side when sleeping

- your urine is dull yellow

- your hair has become thinner and dull

- you combine your age at the time of conception with the number of the month you conceived and the resulting number is odd

- you eat a clove of garlic and don't smell of it

- your previous child's first word was "mama"

- your husband gains weight during your pregnancy

- you were the less aggressive partner during love-making when you conceived

- the highlights in your hair seem to be turning red

- you look a little worn out; your skin breaks out

Add up your "yes" and "no" columns. According to the old wives tales, if you had more "yes's" than "no's" you are more likely having a girl.

Note: these old wives tales only 50% accurate. Keep in mind, whether a woman is carrying the baby "high" or "low" is not dependent on the gender of the baby. The mother's body shape and abdominal muscles are factors involved in the posture of her pregnancy. For example, if a woman has a longer torso, she is more likely to carry her baby lower than a woman who has a shorter torso. However, according to the old wives tales, if a woman is carrying low, she is having a boy. That is simply may not be true if you take into account the woman's body shape.

Chapter 13 - Chinese Baby Gender Calendar

The Chinese Baby Gender Calendar was used in Ancient China for predicting baby gender. It is rumored to have been discovered over 700 years ago in an ancient royal tomb near Beijing, China. Although many people believe that the Chinese Baby Gender Calendar is over 90% accurate for predicting baby gender, it is still only correct half of the time.

The Chinese Baby Gender Calendar is said to have been created due to the strong desire for male babies in the Chinese culture. The males were considered to be more powerful than girls. Therefore, they were able to help out on the farm and contribute financially for the family. Furthermore, the males were able to inherit the family name and property resulting in the continuation of the family name. Females, on the other hand, were more of a liability. The females stayed at home until they got married and then became part of their husband's family. As a result, the female's birth family no longer had control over her life. Essentially, the family was raising a daughter for other people. This was considered "bad business."

Naturally, the Chinese desired to design a technique for predicting baby gender so they could optimize their chances of obtaining the boy they so preferred. Through many years of studying the trends of a woman's age and month at the time of conception, the Chinese Baby Gender Calendar was created.

In order to use the Chinese Baby Gender Calendar for predicting baby gender accurately, it is important to note that the ancient calendar is based on the lunar and solar cycles instead of the solar cycles from our Western culture. As a result, a woman's age at the time of conception and the month she conceived needs to be converted into the lunisolar calendar.

According to the Chinese New Year Calendar, you are already one year old when you are born. Therefore, to determine your lunar age, you would add a year to your current age. However, you may need to add two years depending on the date of the Chinese New Year, which changes every year.

To determine the month of conception according to the lunisolar calendar, you need to compare the Chinese calendar with the Western calendar. The conversion gets complicated due to leap years and other factors involved.

Once your lunar age and the month of conception are established, use the Chinese Baby Gender Calendar below for predicting baby gender. Refer to the mother's age at the time of conception in the left column. Refer to the month of conception in the top row.

(Some information referenced from www.howtodothings.com)

Mother's Age (Lunar)	Month of Conception (Lunar)											
	1st	2nd	3rd	4th	5th	6th	7th	8th	9th	10th	11th	12th
18	G	B	G	B	B	B	B	B	B	B	B	B
19	B	G	B	G	G	B	B	B	B	B	G	G
20	G	B	G	B	B	B	B	B	B	B	B	B
21	B	G	G	G	G	G	G	G	G	G	G	G
22	G	B	B	G	B	G	G	B	G	G	G	G
23	B	B	G	B	B	G	B	G	B	B	B	G
24	B	G	B	B	G	B	B	G	G	G	G	G
25	G	B	B	G	G	B	G	B	B	B	B	B
26	B	G	B	G	G	B	G	B	G	G	G	G
27	G	B	G	B	G	G	B	B	B	B	B	B
28	B	G	B	G	G	G	B	B	B	B	G	G
29	G	B	G	G	B	B	B	B	B	G	G	G
30	B	G	G	G	G	G	G	G	G	G	B	B
31	B	G	B	G	G	G	G	G	G	G	G	B
32	B	G	B	G	G	G	G	G	G	G	G	B
33	G	B	G	B	G	G	G	B	G	G	G	B
34	B	G	B	G	G	G	G	G	G	G	B	B
35	B	B	G	B	G	G	G	B	G	G	B	B
36	G	B	B	G	B	G	G	G	B	B	B	B
37	B	G	B	B	G	B	B	B	G	B	B	B
38	G	B	G	B	B	G	B	B	B	G	B	G
39	B	G	B	B	B	G	G	B	G	B	G	G
40	G	B	G	B	G	B	B	G	B	G	B	G
41	B	G	B	G	B	G	B	B	G	B	G	B
42	G	B	G	B	G	B	G	B	B	G	B	G
43	B	G	B	G	B	G	B	B	B	B	B	B
44	B	B	G	B	B	B	B	B	G	B	G	G
45	G	B	B	G	G	G	B	G	B	G	B	B

Chapter 14 – Semi-Scientific Tests and Methods

There are a few tests and methods rooted in scientific theory that can be used to predict the baby's gender. These semi-scientific tests and methods include the following:

1. The Shettles Method

2. The Heart Rate Test

3. The Fertility Awareness Method.

Shettles Method

Men who play frequent sports or wear tight clothing are said to contribute to predicting baby gender due to the temperature of the scrotum. Since sports and tight clothing constrict the scrotum, the temperature becomes too hot for the sperm. According to the Shettles Method for guessing baby gender, the heat will kill both X (girl) and Y (boy) chromosomes. However, the heat will kill off the less protected, smaller Y chromosomes faster, which means you're more likely to have a girl.

Baby's Heart Rate Test

This semi-scientific method/myth used for guessing baby gender is popular and safe. Essentially, if your doctor tells you that your baby's heart rate is high (over 140 -160 beats per minute), you are having a girl. If your baby's heart rate is below 140 beats per minute, you are having a boy. It is important to keep in mind that scientific studies have failed to prove any correlations between predicting baby gender and heart rate.

Fertility Awareness Method

The gender selection techniques for guessing baby gender uses the timing of intercourse and ovulation. The techniques for predicting baby gender also heavily relies on the different characteristics of sperm (X and Y chromosomes). These concepts of guessing baby gender are the foundation of the Fertility Awareness Method. A fantastic book called *Taking Charge of Your Fertility* by Toni Weschler teaches the concepts of the Fertility Awareness Method.

"Fertility Awareness is a remarkable system of knowledge that uses your two basic fertility signs -waking temperature and cervical fluid- to accurately gauge when you are ovulating. Such critical information serves as a window into your cycle, empowering you to practice effective natural birth control or pregnancy achievement, as well as to enlighten you on the entire array of life's menstrual mysteries. Indeed, charting your cycles with FAM [Fertility Awareness Method] will show you, among other things:

• The difference between perfectly normal, cyclical cervical secretions and true vaginal infections.

• When to expect your next period.

• Whether or not you are even ovulating.

• Whether or not you are pregnant.

• Your true due date, if in fact you are!

It is unfortunate that the Fertility Awareness Method is even referred to as a method, because in reality, it should be seen as a fundamental life skill that all women should learn, just as they are now taught basic feminine hygiene. This is because the practical knowledge women glean from charting their cycles will aid them from puberty to menopause, and all life phases in between" (quote taken from Toni Weschler).

Taking Charge of Your Fertility is an exceptional book that empowers women to learn about their fertility cycle and take control with predicting baby gender. Consequently, women are confident with their body and know when something is wrong because they now know what is supposed to be right. For example, a banker does not learn what the different counterfeit bills look and feel like. There are too many to learn and they are always changing. Instead, the banker learns what an authentic bill looks and feels like so they can quickly pick out the replica bills. Similarly, women need to spend their time learning what is normal about their body As a result, the abnormal symptoms will be easy to identify.

Chapter 15 – Baby Gender Prediction Techniques

When a couple gets pregnant, they are obviously curious to know the gender of the baby. Some couples choose to wait. Others do not. As stated earlier, about 9 out of 10, are interested in predicting baby gender. This group of people would like to predict baby gender in advance for a variety of reasons. One of the more popular reasons is to prepare in advance for the gender specific items that need to be purchased. Even though they may find out the gender of the baby in advance, they usually choose to keep the name a secret so there is some element of surprise.

These pregnant couples that want to predict baby gender in advance find out through an ultrasound at about 20 weeks pregnant. However, what if there was a way to predict baby gender BEFORE even getting pregnant? Using gender selection techniques for predicting baby gender can be used to greatly increase the likelihood of achieving a particular gender. Although nature will always take its course, we can use the predicting baby gender techniques to tip the scales in our favour.

In order to practice the gender selection techniques for predicting baby gender, several concepts need to be understood to influence the baby's gender. These concepts include:

1. Male Sperm Characteristics

2. Intercourse and Ovulation Timing

3. Female Diet

4. Female Orgasms

5. Sex Positions

6. Ovulation Predictor Kits

Male Sperm: X and Y Chromosomes

Before trying to get pregnant, it is important to know the characteristics of the male's sperm. Between the male and female, it is the male who determines the gender of baby during pregnancy. The male sperm is made up of two chromosomes: X and Y. The X chromosomes produce girls and the Y chromosomes produce boys. The X chromosomes are larger, slower and live longer. The Y chromosomes are smaller, faster and die quicker.

Intercourse and Ovulation Timing

Considering the information about the two chromosomes in male sperm, the timing of intercourse and ovulation become critical in predicting baby gender.

If you want a girl...engage in intercourse two to three days before ovulation begins. Sperm lives up to five days in the female body. The extra days will give time for the female sperm to beat the male sperm and wait for the arrival of the egg.

If you want a boy...engage in intercourse one day before or the day of ovulation. As a result, the male sperm will reach the egg before the female sperm.

Female Acidity and Diet

The PH balance inside of females can dictate gender of baby during pregnancy. The more acidic the environment is, the more likely to conceive a girl. Conversely, the more alkaline the environment is, the more likely to conceive a boy. Therefore, the female diet can influence the PH balance and affect predicting baby gender. If a girl is desired, the woman should choose foods such as apples, broccoli and fish.

Female Orgasms

In conjunction with the PH balance is the opportunity for a woman to orgasm. Surprisingly, whether or not a woman has an orgasm during sexual intercourse can affect gender of baby during pregnancy. When a woman orgasms, the PH balance becomes more alkaline, which is conducive to a boy. Therefore, the woman should avoid having an orgasm altogether. Conversely, if a boy is desired, the woman should have an orgasm just before or at the same time as her male partner.

Sex Positions

Believe it or not, the sexual position used during intercourse can influence gender of baby during pregnancy. If hopes are for a girl, focus on shallow penetration positions like the "missionary position". This position will deposit the sperm away from the cervix, therefore giving an advantage to the slower, longer living female sperm. Deep penetration positions, such as rear entry or "doggy-style", can result in a boy. Essentially, the sperm is delivered right to the doorstep of the cervix so the lazy male sperm has less of a distance to travel.

Ovulation Predictor Kits

In order for predicting baby gender to be even possible, a woman must be ovulating to have a chance of getting pregnant. Purchasing an ovulation predictor kit is a great way to know if you are ovulating or not. There are cheaper ways of tracking your ovulation by simply using a basal body thermometer, a pencil and a calendar.

Chapter 16 – The Female Predicts Baby Gender

It is usually widely accepted that the male partner determines the sex of the baby based on the X and Y chromosomes in the sperm. When the sperm reach the ovum (female egg), either the X chromosome penetrates the ovum and confirms a baby girl. Or the Y chromosome fertilizes the ovum and confirms a baby boy. However, the ovum may have a larger role to play in the determination of the baby's gender.

Science is discovering that the ovum can actually pick and choose which chromosome it will allow to fertilize itself. This research reveals that the ovum is not passive in accepting whichever sperm is able to penetrate the cell membrane, called the zona pellucida. In fact, the zona pellucida can change its chemical composition to attract or repel either X or Y chromosomes. Therefore, regardless of which chromosomes are predominately around the ovum, the ovum has the final say in which one it will accept.

Conclusion

Thank you again for purchasing *"How to Predict Your Baby Gender: Guide to Fertility and Achieving the Baby Gender of Your Dreams."*

I hope this book was able to provide you with practical strategies for helping you get pregnant faster and predicting your baby's gender.

The next step is to go to it and have some fun! Try to relax and not get too uptight with the planning. Stress can definitely debilitate your chances of getting pregnant.

Finally, if you enjoyed this book and found it meaningful, please take the time to share your thoughts and post a positive review on Amazon. I greatly appreciate your time and effort.

I would love for you to share your experiences, stories and encouragements with me. My email address is kristinaducloskindle@gmail.com

I sincerely thank you for taking the time to read my book. I truly hope the best for you and your baby making journey.

In addition, please remember to check out our Facebook page in order to find other resources and upcoming promotions:

https://www.facebook.com/joypublishing

With gratitude,

Kristina Duclos

Preview of "Diaper Free Baby Guide: Elimination Communication Strategies for Quicker and Healthier Potty Training Before 18 Months"

Introduction

I want to thank you and congratulate you for purchasing the book, *"Diaper Free Baby Guide: Elimination Communication Strategies for Quicker and Healthier Potty Training Before 18 Months."*

This book contains proven steps and strategies on how to teach your child natural potty training quickly and without the use of diapers!

Are you having a hard time introducing your child to the proper use of the toilet? You're not alone! Millions of parents are having a hard time switching their babies from diapers to regular toilet use. Using this eBook however, you'll learn exactly how to approach the problem with minimum fuss from the child. Even at just a few months old, this book will be able to walk you through natural toilet training and have your toddler fully trained before s/he hits 18 months!

Thanks again for purchasing this book, I hope you enjoy it! Please take some time to stop by and LIKE our Facebook page:

https://www.facebook.com/joypublishing

With gratitude,

Kristina Duclos

Chapter 1: What Is Elimination Communication?

Elimination Communication is a potty-training system that has been popular with parents for a number of years now. Although still not firmly latched in the mainstream, there's no question that Elimination Communication is getting attention from many parents, especially those who want to tackle and get over potty training early and quickly.

The system is basically a potty-training method that starts early – perhaps just a few days after the child is born. The gist of it is being able to anticipate the baby's need to eliminate and providing them with the right environment to do the deed - usually the toilet.

How It Works

Simply put, parents make use of different signals, intuition, cues, and timing to find out whether their baby would eliminate or not. Once these cues are noticed, the parent can do whatever it is that needs to be done to prepare the child for elimination. In most cases, the child is held over the toilet, allowing for an easy clean up for the parent. As the child grows up, s/he becomes more and more used to the routine, making it easier for parents to instruct them in the "adult" way of going to the potty.

How It Started

Parents in developed countries usually make use of diapers for their children, allowing them to conveniently remove the item and throw it away. However, undeveloped countries approach potty training in a different manner – as ascertained by Ingrid Bauer.

In her book *Diaper Free! The Gentle Wisdom of Natural Infant Hygiene* released in 2001, Bauer talks about the natural hygiene she witnessed in Africa and employed the same tactics with her children. According to her, there were very little elimination accidents even as parents carried their babies with them every day in a sling.

Of course, Bauer's book isn't exactly the first method to approach "natural" potty training. However, it seems to be the one with the most impact in the modern world.

When to Start

As already mentioned, natural infant hygiene is something you can start just a few weeks after the baby is born. However, this might be a little uncomfortable for you, especially since at this stage, the child is a bit more delicate. If you're wary of starting EC a few days after birth, you can try waiting for the 3rd month or at anytime you're happy with the child's movement control. You can simply use the first few months for information as you understand your child's bowel movements and the signals they often use.

Note though that you should NEVER wait until the child is 5 months. Although the baby is still young at this point, a diaper-filled life gets them accustomed to the sensation, therefore making it harder to train them using EC.

Now that you've gotten the gist of Elimination Communication, it's time to talk about its many benefits and how you can apply the same technique with your kids. Prior to proceeding however, it's best to first clear up some terminology issues. For the purpose of this book, Elimination Communication can be used interchangeably with EC, natural infant hygiene, nappy free and infant potty training.

Check out the rest of "Diaper Free Baby Guide: Elimination Communication Strategies for Quicker and Healthier Potty Training Before 18 Months" on Amazon

Or go to: http://amzn.to/1kPRAC8

One Last Thing...

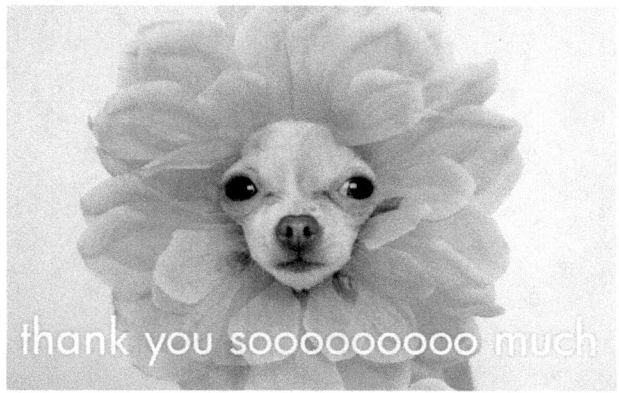

thank you soooooooooo much

Source: Wikipedia

If you believe that this book is worth sharing, would you please take the time to let others know how it affected your life? If it turns out to make a difference in the lives of others, they will be forever grateful to you, as will I.